VALERIAN ROOT FOR BEGINNERS

Unlocking Peaceful Sleep, The Holistic Guide To Valerian Root For Deep Rest, Stress Relief, And Relaxation

Georgette Lockett

© [2023] [Georgette Lockett]

All rights reserved. No part of this publication may be reproduced, distributed, or transmitted in any form or by any means, including photocopying, recording, or other electronic or mechanical methods, without the prior written permission of the publisher, except in the case of brief quotations embodied in critical reviews and certain other noncommercial uses permitted by copyright law.

DISCLAIMER

The author of this book is not affiliated, associated, endorsed, sponsored, or approved by any company or individual. The views and opinions expressed in this book are solely those of the author and do not necessarily reflect the official policy or position of any entity.

The author hereby disclaims any relationship, collaboration, or partnership with any company or individual mentioned in this book. Any references to products, services, or individuals are provided for informational purposes only and should not be construed as an endorsement or recommendation.

Readers are advised to exercise their own judgment and discretion when applying the information provided in this book. The author shall not be held responsible for any actions taken by readers based on the content of this book.

This book is intended for general informational purposes only, and the author makes no representations or warranties of any kind, express or implied, about the completeness, accuracy, reliability, suitability, or availability of the information contained herein. Any reliance on the information in this book is at the reader's own risk.

The author reserves the right to update, change, or modify any information in this book without notice. It is the responsibility of the reader to verify any information before taking any actions based on the content of this book.

By reading this book, the reader acknowledges and agrees to the terms of this disclaimer.

Table of Contents

INTRODUCTION 8

Overview Of Valerian Root 8

Historical Background...................................9

Importance In Traditional Medicine 9

CHAPTER 1 12

Botanical Profile 12

Taxonomy And Classification......................12

Morphological Features 12

Geographic Distribution 13

CHAPTER 2 16

Chemical Composition 16

Key Compounds And Constituents 16

Valerenic Acid 17

Isovaleric Acid...17

Essential Oils 18

CHAPTER 3 20

Pharmacology...20

Mechanisms Of Action 20

Interaction With Gaba Receptors 20

Effects On The Central Nervous System 21

Other Pharmacological Actions.........................21

CHAPTER 4 24

Medicinal Uses 24

Sleep Disorders And Insomnia 24

Anxiety And Stress Management 24

Muscle Relaxation 25

Other Therapeutic Applications 25

CHAPTER 5 28

Clinical Studies And Research 28

Overview Of Relevant Studies 28

Efficacy In Sleep Disorders 28

2. Sleep Patterns: 29

3. Anxiety-Related Sleep Disorders: 29

Safety And Side Effects 30

CHAPTER 6 32

Forms Of Administration 32

Herbal Tea..32

Tinctures 33

Capsules And Tablets 33

Topical Applications 34

CHAPTER 7 36

Dosage And Guidelines....................................36

Recommended Dosages 36

Considerations For Specific Conditions..............37

• Insomnia and Sleep Disorders: 37

• Anxiety and Stress: 37

• Other Medical problems: 38

Potential Interactions And Contraindications 38

CHAPTER 8 40

Cultivation And Harvesting 40

Growing Conditions 40

Harvesting Practices...........................40

Sustainability Considerations 41

CHAPTER 9 42

Quality Control And Standardization 42

Importance Of Quality Assurance 42

Standardization Of Valerian Products...............42

Regulatory Guidelines 43

CHAPTER 10 46

Future Perspectives 46

Ongoing Research..............................46

Potential Innovations 47

Emerging Trends 48

Conclusion 49

THE END 53

INTRODUCTION

Valerian root, obtained from the Valeriana officinalis plant, has a rich historical heritage firmly anchored in traditional medicine. This perennial blooming plant, native to Europe and parts of Asia, has been famous for its medical virtues for ages. Its name is said to stem from the Latin word "valere," meaning "to be strong or healthy," reflecting its ancient usage as a treatment for many diseases.

Overview Of Valerian Root

Valerian root is generally renowned for its possible relaxing and sedative properties, typically employed to manage sleep difficulties, anxiety, and anxiety. The root includes a range of chemicals, including valerenic acid, valerian, and several alkaloids, which are considered to contribute to its medicinal benefits.

These substances interact with neurotransmitters in the brain, notably gamma-aminobutyric acid (GABA), a crucial neurotransmitter involved in controlling anxiety and fostering relaxation.

Historical Background

Valerian root has a long and rich history stretching back to ancient civilizations. Its usage may be dated back as early as ancient Greece and Rome when it was utilized for its alleged medical effects. Valerian's relaxing effects were identified and exploited by herbalists and healers throughout the centuries. Its usage grew prevalent throughout Europe during the medieval era and continued to gain favor into the Renaissance.

Importance In Traditional Medicine

In traditional medicine systems such as Ayurveda and Traditional Chinese Medicine (TCM), valerian root was highly appreciated for its soothing and relaxing qualities. It was widely given as a cure for sleeplessness, anxiety, headaches, and many stress-related illnesses. The plant was also believed good for resolving stomach disorders and muscular relaxation.

The prominence of valerian root in traditional medical systems refers to its perceived effectiveness and the observations made by practitioners over generations. Its integration into numerous herbal cures and formulations emphasizes its relevance as a natural medicinal agent.

Across diverse cultures and ages, valerian root has had a steady reputation for its capacity to induce relaxation, reduce anxiety, and enhance sleep quality. Its historical use has opened the path for current scientific study and confirmation of its pharmacological qualities, resulting in its widespread use in contemporary herbal medicine and supplements.

CHAPTER 1

Botanical Profile

Taxonomy And Classification

Valerian Root, technically known as Valeriana officinalis, belongs to the family Caprifoliaceae. This perennial blooming plant has a lengthy history of therapeutic usage extending back millennia. The genus Valeriana has approximately 250 species, with Valeriana officinalis being the most frequently known and exploited species for its medicinal benefits.

Morphological Features

Valerian is distinguished by its sturdy, upright, hollow stems that may grow up to 5 feet in height. The plant boasts complex, fern-like leaves separated into smaller leaflets, frequently with serrated edges.

The leaves exude a unique odor that may be fairly intense when crushed or injured.

The root system is the major focus for therapeutic reasons. Valerian's root is twisted and knotted, like a cluster of ropes, and has a strong, earthy fragrance that some find unpleasant. The roots are gathered for their therapeutic components.

Geographic Distribution

Valerian is indigenous to Europe and portions of Asia, although it has become naturalized in numerous places worldwide. It thrives in temperate temperatures and is typically found in wet or marshy locations, along riverbanks, and in meadows. Cultivation has expanded its reach beyond its original habitats, and it's currently grown in various nations for its therapeutic benefits.

Throughout history, this herb has been treasured for its possible soothing and relaxing qualities. Its botanical traits and unique chemicals make it a topic of interest in pharmacology and traditional medicinal practices.

CHAPTER 2

Chemical Composition

Valerian root, formally known as Valeriana officinalis, is recognized for its unique chemical makeup, which adds to its medicinal effects. This chapter digs into the essential elements and ingredients that make Valerian Root a beneficial plant in different traditional and contemporary therapeutic applications.

Key Compounds And Constituents

Valerian root includes a varied variety of chemicals that contribute to its pharmacological actions. Among them, valepotriates, alkaloids, flavonoids, and essential oils are some of the most prominent. Each of these components has a part in the overall effectiveness of Valerian Root as an herbal treatment.

Valerenic Acid

One of the key and most investigated components in Valerian Root is valerenic acid. This sesquiterpene is considered to be responsible for the anxiolytic (anxiety-reducing) and calming actions of the plant. Valerenic acid interacts with the GABAergic system, which is important in the control of anxiety and sleep.

Isovaleric Acid

Isovaleric acid is another key component discovered in Valerian roots. It adds to the unique odor of the plant. Isovaleric acid is thought to improve the sedative characteristics of Valerian Root and is regarded to be one of the components responsible for its soothing effects on the central nervous system.

Essential Oils

Essential oils contained in Valerian Root, notably bornyl acetate, pinene, and camphene, contribute to the overall biological activity of the plant. These oils are recognized for their capacity to promote relaxation and reduce stress. The combination of these essential oils with other substances generates a synergistic effect, improving the herb's medicinal potential.

Understanding the chemical makeup of Valerian Root is vital for appreciating its methods of action and the spectrum of therapeutic advantages it provides. The following chapters will further investigate how these components interact with the body, impacting numerous physiological processes and making Valerian Root an important plant in the domain of natural medicine.

CHAPTER 3

Pharmacology

Mechanisms Of Action

Valerian Root's pharmacological efficacy is mostly related to its wide mix of bioactive chemicals. Its modes of action entail the regulation of neurotransmitters and receptors, especially gamma-aminobutyric acid (GABA), the principal inhibitory neurotransmitter in the brain.

Interaction With Gaba Receptors

Valerian's interaction with GABA receptors is important to its pharmacological actions. Compounds like valerenic acid prevent the breakdown of GABA in the brain, resulting in higher GABA levels. Valerian's influence on GABA receptors may generate a relaxing effect, increasing relaxation and perhaps assisting sleep.

Effects On The Central Nervous System

Valerian's effects on the central nervous system are diverse. It impacts several neurotransmitter systems beyond GABA, including serotonin and norepinephrine. By regulating these neurotransmitters, it may contribute to their anxiolytic (anxiety-reducing) and sedative qualities.

The chemical isovaleric acid also appears to have a role in its soothing effects. Though its specific processes are not explained, isovaleric acid possibly adds to Valerian's sedative properties.

Other Pharmacological Actions

In addition to its action on neurotransmitters, Valerian has anti-inflammatory and antioxidant qualities, which may contribute to its overall effects on the body. According to research, these qualities may help to preserve the neurological system and reduce oxidative stress.

Valerian has also been studied for its ability to treat illnesses such as sleeplessness, anxiety, and stress. While additional study is needed, early results suggest that it might be used as an alternative or supplemental treatment for various disorders.

Understanding Valerian Root pharmacology entails a complicated interaction of its many components and their effects on diverse physiological pathways. While it shows promise, more comprehensive clinical trials are required to fully clarify its processes and therapeutic potential across a wide range of health issues.

This chapter looks into Valerian Root's extensive pharmacological properties, revealing light on its varied impacts on the body's physiological systems, notably the central nervous system, as well as providing insight into its possible therapeutic uses.

CHAPTER 4

Medicinal Uses

Sleep Disorders And Insomnia

One of the most well-known and widely researched applications of valerian root is its ability to help sleep and treat sleep disorders. Its sedative qualities are due to its interaction with GABA receptors in the brain, which promotes relaxation and may improve sleep quality. Its usefulness in lowering the time it takes to fall asleep and enhancing sleep duration without the grogginess associated with other pharmacological sleep aids has been shown in studies.

Anxiety And Stress Management

Valerian root has also been used to treat anxiety and stress symptoms. Its interaction with GABA receptors may contribute to its anxiolytic effects, assisting in the relaxation of the mind and the reduction of sensations of anxiety. While not as powerful as certain prescription drugs, it is often seen as a gentler, natural option with fewer side effects.

Muscle Relaxation

Aside from its ability to improve sleep and reduce anxiety, valerian root is well-known for its muscle-relaxing qualities. Individuals suffering from muscular tension, cramping, or overall pain may benefit from this effect. Its soothing effect on the central nervous system aids in the relief of muscle tension, making it effective for people experiencing minor muscular pain.

Other Therapeutic Applications

Valerian root has also been studied for additional purposes such as menstrual cramp treatment, migraine management, and digestive disorders, however, more study is required to confirm its usefulness clearly in these areas.

Because of its flexibility in treating several aspects of sleep and relaxation, valerian root is a popular option among those looking for natural therapies for sleep disorders, anxiety, and moderate stress.

The many uses of valerian root for sleep, anxiety, and muscular tension highlight its promise as a natural, holistic medicine. When contemplating its usage for therapeutic reasons, it is important to consider individual variances in reaction as well as possible interactions with other drugs or health problems.

CHAPTER 5

Clinical Studies And Research

Overview Of Relevant Studies

Numerous research studies have been conducted to investigate the medicinal effects of Valerian Root, with a special emphasis on its potential in the management of different illnesses, mainly sleep problems and anxiety. The study of its effectiveness often focuses on its sedative and anxiolytic effects.

Efficacy In Sleep Disorders

Valerian Root has received a lot of attention for its usefulness in enhancing sleep quality and treating insomnia. Research has shown that it can reduce sleep latency (the time it takes to fall asleep) and improve sleep quality without the side effects associated with many other sleep aids.

1. Valerian's usefulness in treating insomnia has been studied in many clinical investigations. Although individual reactions may vary, the findings show that it may enhance sleep quality and shorten the time it takes to fall asleep. The processes behind these benefits are most likely due to its interaction with GABA receptors in the brain, which promotes relaxation and sleep induction without causing the sedation observed with pharmacological sleep aids.

2. **Sleep Patterns:** Research has also looked at Valerian's influence on sleep architecture, specifically its capacity to improve deep sleep (slow-wave sleep) and regulate sleep cycles. This is especially crucial when it comes to treating sleep disruptions and developing a more restorative sleep pattern.

3. **Anxiety-Related Sleep Disorders:** Valerian Root has also been studied in situations when sleep disorders are associated with anxiety. Its anxiolytic characteristics may contribute to its effectiveness in

increasing sleep quality by reducing anxiety, encouraging relaxation, and therefore allowing for better sleep.

Safety And Side Effects

While Valerian Root is usually regarded as safe for short-term usage, it is critical to analyze its safety profile, particularly in terms of possible adverse effects and interactions.

1. In clinical investigations, Valerian Root was shown to have little side effects when used for a short period. However, long-term safety evidence is still scarce, necessitating vigilance in extended or high-dose use. Its safety during pregnancy, breastfeeding, and in pediatric populations also needs to be investigated further.

2. When side effects are reported, they are often moderate and may include gastrointestinal disorders, headaches, dizziness, and daytime sleepiness.

These events, however, are rather rare.

3. Valerian Root may interact with several drugs, including sedatives, antidepressants, and chemicals that influence the central nervous system. Individuals taking other drugs should thus check their healthcare professionals before using Valerian to prevent possible problems.

Valerian Root shows potential as a natural treatment for sleep disorders and moderate anxiety. Clinical investigations have shown its ability to enhance sleep quality and treat insomnia, owing mostly to its interactions with the GABA system. However, further study is required to confirm its long-term safety profile, especially in different demographics and possible drug interactions.

The results of this chapter highlight the relevance of Valerian Root as an alternative or additional strategy for treating sleep problems and anxiety, with more research into its effectiveness, safety, and proper dosage recommendations required.

CHAPTER 6

Forms Of Administration

Valerian Root, which is recognized for its sedative and anxiolytic characteristics, is taken in a variety of forms, each customized to personal preferences and desired results.

Herbal Tea

Making Valerian Root tea is one of the most ancient and traditional ways of ingestion. This method is steeping dried Valerian roots in hot water. However, some people may find the taste unpleasant because of its strong, earthy flavor and pungent odor. However, this procedure is simple and provides a natural manner to take Valerian Root, allowing for the steady release of its medicinal chemicals.

Tinctures

Tinctures are extremely concentrated versions of Valerian Root that are frequently alcohol-based preparations. These solutions are made by soaking the root in alcohol or an alcohol-water combination and allowing the active ingredients to dissolve. Tinctures are often easier to use than teas and provide a more strong dose. Their liquid state also provides for faster absorption and speedier activation inside the body.

Capsules And Tablets

Capsules and pills are a practical option for people who dislike the taste of Valerian. These products include powdered Valerian Root or standardized extracts, which allow for exact dose management. They are often found at health food shops and pharmacies. This approach is appropriate for those who want the advantages of Valerian Root without the flavor or texture that comes with other versions.

Topical Applications

Valerian Root essential oils and extracts are occasionally utilized topically, despite their rarity. Valerian Root creams, oils, and ointments are applied to the skin. These applications, according to supporters, may aid with localized pain or muscular relaxation. However, as compared to oral treatment, information on the effectiveness of topical Valerian formulations is sparse.

Each mode of administration has various benefits, and the decision is often influenced by personal preferences, convenience, desired potency, and therapeutic efficacy. When taking Valerian Root with other drugs or supplements, it is important to consider dose, product quality, and any interactions or contraindications.

Understanding the different modes of administration allows users to choose the best technique for their unique requirements, assuring an effective and tailored approach to consuming Valerian Root for its possible health advantages.

CHAPTER 7

Dosage And Guidelines

Valerian root has a rich history that is strongly anchored in traditional medicine and is still relevant in modern healthcare procedures. Let us now look at Chapter 7, which focuses on dose, recommendations, and concerns for its usage.

Recommended Dosages

The proper dose for valerian root depends on several variables, including the formulation, intended usage (for anxiety, sleeplessness, etc.), individual sensitivity, and the potency of the particular product. For dry herbal medicines, dosages vary from 300 milligrams to 900 milligrams, administered 30 minutes to two hours before bedtime to improve sleep quality. A common dosage of liquid extracts is 1-2 tablespoons before sleep. However, depending on the concentration of the product, these dosages may change.

The dose for anxiety may also vary, frequently falling within the same range but being taken many times during the day. Individual response and clinical trials are critical in establishing the most effective dosage.

Considerations For Specific Conditions

• **Insomnia and Sleep Disorders:** Valerian root is well-known for its ability to promote better sleep. It is important to remember, however, that its effects might take time to develop. It may take several weeks of consistent usage to detect changes in sleep quality.

• **Anxiety and Stress:** Valerian root's anxiolytic qualities may help with anxiety and stress management. However, it may not have the same instant effects as medications.

For acute anxiety, various therapies may be required at first, and valerian root might be taken as a supplement.

• **Other Medical problems:** People who have pre-existing medical problems or are on medication should see a doctor before using valerian root since it may interfere with some drugs or worsen certain health issues.

Potential Interactions And Contraindications

The interactions of Valerian root with other drugs or pharmaceuticals may reduce its effectiveness or cause health hazards. It has the potential to exacerbate the effects of other drugs that cause excessive sedation or sleepiness, especially when used with substances that also influence the central nervous system.

Individuals with liver illness or damage should also exercise caution since there have been rare occurrences of liver toxicity linked to valerian root supplementation.

Using valerian root when pregnant or nursing is typically discouraged owing to a lack of data about its safety during these times.

Valerian root is not suggested for use in children under the age of three, and owing to insufficient research on its benefits and safety in these groups, care should be given when contemplating its usage in children or teenagers.

Understanding these dose parameters, unique considerations, and possible interactions is critical for using valerian root as an herbal supplement safely and effectively. Before starting any new supplement regimen, always speak with a healthcare practitioner to verify it corresponds with specific health requirements and prevents any issues.

CHAPTER 8

Cultivation And Harvesting

Growing Conditions

Valerian, formally known as Valeriana officinalis, grows best in temperate areas, preferring wet, well-drained soil and light shade. Its cultivation generally starts with the division of seeds or roots. The plant's life cycle lasts two years, and the root is the main therapeutic component. The plant develops its vegetative components during the first year, while the root system expands significantly during the second year.

Harvesting Practices

Valerian root is best harvested during its dormancy, which occurs in October when the aerial portions have withered back. To maintain the roots' purity and therapeutic power, they are carefully dug up.

After harvest, the roots are cleaned, chopped, and dried to decrease moisture content and ensure quality and lifespan.

Sustainability Considerations

Because of rising demand and habitat degradation, sustainable farming procedures for Valerian are critical. Sustainable harvesting practices seek to protect natural populations and biodiversity. Initiatives support responsible sourcing by encouraging farmers to use ethical practices such as crop rotation and organic farming. This contributes to the plant's medical potency while reducing environmental impact.

To ensure the supply of this unique botanical treatment, it is critical to balance the rising demand for Valerian Root with sustainable farming techniques.

CHAPTER 9

Quality Control And Standardization

Importance Of Quality Assurance

Importance of Quality Assurance Valerian Root's efficacy and safety are heavily reliant on the product's quality. As an herbal treatment, quality assurance begins with cultivation and continues through extraction, formulation, and packing. Quality control ensures that the finished product includes the intended active ingredients in sufficient quantities to provide consistent and reliable results.

Standardization Of Valerian Products

Valerian Product Standardization Ensures that specified components or compounds, frequently the active substances responsible for medicinal benefits, are present in consistent and quantifiable levels in each batch of herbal products. This largely includes substances such as valerenic acid, isovaleric acid, and specific essential oils in the case of Valerian Root. Standardization helps anticipate the effectiveness and safety of a product, enabling customers to make educated judgments.

Regulatory Guidelines

Regulatory authorities across the globe have varying standards and policies for herbal supplements, including Valerian Root products. These rules are intended to protect consumers by ensuring product uniformity and correct labeling. To maintain quality and safety requirements in the manufacturing process, manufacturers must follow Good Manufacturing Practices (GMP). These requirements vary by area, with some governments enforcing stricter laws than others.

To ensure quality control and uniformity, thorough testing for purity, potency, and contaminants is required. To detect and quantify active chemicals while monitoring for impurities, pesticides, heavy metals, and microbial contamination, several analytical methods such as High-Performance Liquid Chromatography (HPLC) and Gas Chromatography-Mass Spectrometry (GC-MS) are used.

Additionally, standardized extracts or formulations are intended to give constant doses, enabling healthcare practitioners and consumers to correctly assess consumption and anticipated effects. This consistency is essential for both safety and effectiveness, particularly when Valerian Root is used therapeutically.

Overall, strict quality control procedures, standardization processes, and regulatory compliance are critical in guaranteeing the safety, effectiveness, and trustworthiness of Valerian Root products on the market. This certification benefits consumers by providing access to high-quality herbal supplements with predictable effects and reduced health hazards.

CHAPTER 10

Future Perspectives

Valerian Root has a long history and many uses, but its journey does not stop there or even in the present. Looking forward, some intriguing opportunities and possibilities might improve our knowledge and use of this herbal treatment.

Ongoing Research

The scientific community is still researching Valerian Root's pharmacology and therapeutic potential. Ongoing study strives to learn more about its active chemicals, how they interact in the body, and the entire range of its physiological effects. Researchers are using advanced approaches to investigate the molecular principles behind Valerian Root's pharmacological activities as technology progresses.

Several research are being conducted to investigate new aspects of Valerian Root's effect on the central nervous system. This involves looking into possible synergies with other plants or drugs, as well as learning how Valerian interacts with particular neurotransmitter systems beyond its well-known impact on GABA receptors.

Potential Innovations

Future Valerian Root use may go beyond typical herbal preparations. To improve bioavailability and effectiveness, researchers are experimenting with new formulations and delivery modalities. This might result in the creation of standardized extracts or pharmaceutical formulations with accurate dosages and consistent therapeutic effects.

There is potential for breakthroughs in breeding procedures to enhance the amount of important chemicals like valerenic acid in the cultivation domain.

This might result in Valerian plants with increased therapeutic characteristics, resulting in more effective and dependable products.

Emerging Trends

Valerian Root is expected to be a topic of debate in conversations about natural treatments for stress, anxiety, and sleep difficulties. Valerian Root may see an increase in interest and usage as a supplementary or alternative treatment as knowledge of holistic health practices grows.

Furthermore, as sustainability becomes more important in herbal therapy, there may be a movement toward responsible growing and harvesting procedures. Demand for ethically produced, ecologically friendly Valerian goods may drive business improvements, advocating a balance between providing consumer demands and protecting the ecosystems that sustain Valerian Root's development.

To summarize, Valerian Root's future shows promise in terms of greater scientific findings, novel uses, and heightened awareness of sustainable behaviors. Valerian Root serves as a tribute to the continuous importance of ancient herbal knowledge, along with the thrill of current study and future possibilities, as we navigate this changing world.

Conclusion

Valerian root, technically known as Valeriana officinalis, has a long history that is profoundly entwined with traditional medicine. This plant has been revered for generations for its ability to treat numerous diseases and induce calm. It has been respected for millennia in traditional medical systems, notably in Europe and Asia, for its soothing and healing powers.

The chemical makeup of valerian root takes center stage in Chapter 2. The roots contain a wide range of chemicals, but the most important ones are valeric acid, isovaleric acid, and essential oils. Valerenic acid, in particular, is important in its pharmacological effects, regulating how it interacts with the neurological system.

In Chapter 3, we look at the pharmacology of the valerian root to learn more about its methods of action. It mainly functions as a moderate sedative and anxiolytic drug by interacting with GABA receptors in the brain. Valerian root has soothing effects on the central nervous system by regulating these receptors, providing relief from stress and anxiety, and maybe promoting sleep.

Dosage and recommendations, as outlined in Chapter 7, are critical considerations. Dosages are recommended depending on the intended usage, and individual tolerance and product potency differences must be considered.

Understanding unique concerns for different illnesses, possible drug interactions, and contraindications is critical for safe and successful administration.

Chapter 8 discusses cultivation and harvesting methods. Valerian root grows best under specified circumstances, preferring damp, temperate regions. Because of the rising demand for this plant, sustainable harvesting procedures are critical to guaranteeing its supply while protecting habitats.

Chapter 10's exploration of future possibilities offers an interesting world. Ongoing study continues to unearth novel aspects of the pharmacology of valerian root, either revealing new medicinal uses or improving established ones. Innovations in extraction processes, formulations, and administration modalities may improve its effectiveness and accessibility, allowing it to be used more widely.

In conclusion, summing these chapters illustrates the diverse character of the valerian root. Its chemical ingredients, pharmacological activities, dose recommendations, cultivation, and prospects all highlight its importance in the fields of wellness and herbal therapy. Reflecting on its historical usage and current relevance underlines its importance as a natural cure that provides relaxation as well as possible therapeutic effects.

THE END